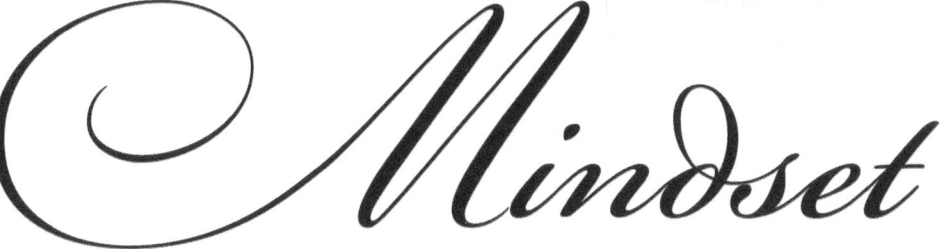

Mindset

Healthy Response
The Attitude Solution for
Permanent Weight Loss

GARY BRISKER

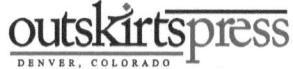

outskirtspress

DENVER, COLORADO

Table of Contents

Introduction

What would happen if you tried to drive a car with one wheel horribly out of alignment? What if two tires were straight, one aimed slightly to the right and the other to the left? The car wouldn't get very far, would it?

Yet that's how most of us live our lives because we don't maintain a healthy balance between the four categories that lead us to a fulfilling and holistic life: nutritional, physical, emotional and spiritual. After more than thirty years and 50,000 hours of successful one-on-one nutritional counseling, I've discovered that fad diets and trendy exercise programs lead primarily to a roller-coaster of weight losses and weight gains. People get in and out of shape because they haven't taken the time to balance the four components of their lives. We may work out, but we don't eat right. Or we get so hung up on *making* a living that we stop living. Without having all four elements of your life in alignment, you'll never be able to stay on the road that leads to your dreams being realized – whether it's losing weight, having a better body, getting in shape, finding a better job, having a fulfilling relationship, or just waking up every morning with a sense of hope instead of despair. Without proper balance, you'll eventually break down, just like the car with the wheels out of alignment.

We all know that in our society size matters: the size of our bank account, the size of our house, the size of a dress, the size of the pants we wear. We're judged every day. The purpose of this book is to help you develop the habits necessary to have a body that makes you proud. In turn, your self-esteem, self-respect and self-confidence will make you feel better about all aspects of your life. There are emotional, physical, spiritual and nutritional formulas in this book that will change your life forever.

The bottom line to remember is this: NO DIET WORKS. Diets end. You have to make a lifestyle change and an on-going emotional commitment to yourself that you will follow the nutritional plan outlined in this book. It's not about food deprivation. You can eat three meals a day and adhere to the various healthy responses for Weight Loss that you will learn about later.

I took an overweight man and woman on "Weight-Loss Wednesday," a morning TV spot I do for the CB affiliate in Phoenix, and put them on my nutritional plan. They had to weigh in live on TV every week – it wasn't a doctored before-and-after picture like you see in magazine ads and in other books – and in 13 weeks, the woman lost more than 30 pounds and the man lost 46 and they kept the weight off. If you learn to make the same emotional commitment to yourself and follow this plan, it will be the jump-start to your new healthy life, too.

The first thing you have to ask yourself before embarking on any journey toward self-improvement is, "Am I in holistic alignment?" Here's what you need to understand about each category in order to find out:

- **Nutritional.** Eighty percent of what you look like and how you feel is what you eat. You can walk to the moon and back and eat for 30 minutes for immediate gratification and the food will negate all that exercise. But whether you exercise or not, it's not going to eliminate certain cancers that are caused by preservatives, additives, emulsifiers, solidifiers, dyes and chemicals in the foods we eat. And if you don't consume the right foods, you can exercise until the cows come home and you're still going to jiggle on the beach.

- **Physical**. What are your hobbies? What do you do to keep moving and feeling alive? What activities excite you? Are you an active participant in those activities? We're a nation of watchers – athletes, actors and singers – when we should be participants. Be a doer, not just a dreamer. It's time to stop watching and start doing.

- **Emotional.** You have to strip away the things that hold you back and nurture the things that make you feel good. Sentences, words and contact with other people can either weigh you down or make you feel so powerful that you think you could fly like Superman. Don't let anyone rain on your parade, tell you that you can't do something, or set limits that will stifle you or make you feel like you're in a rut. Become self-sufficient and independent enough that you don't need another person to survive, but rather you want to share things with other people in order to thrive.

- **Spiritual**. Is there purpose in your life? It doesn't have to be religious, but it can be. It can be a job that fulfills you, volunteer work, or even a pet you care for. But there has to be some purpose to life that will keep you from sitting comatose in front of the TV, feeding your face and wasting your precious time on Earth.

The four categories that make up a holistic life must be in symmetry for you to be the person you dream of being. you can be the most religiously and spiritually fulfilled person in the world, but if you go home and polish off a dozen Krispie Kreme donuts that go straight to your thighs, the physical and nutritional parts of your life will be out of balance. Or you can work out six hours a day and eat healthy, but if you have no other purpose, you will be the best-looking depressed person on the planet.

In this book, we will walk together through a series of steps that will help you discover six building blocks, centered around the four life-balance elements. These steps will lead you to a holistic life and create a ring of strength or life preserver to rescue you from the sea of sorrow that tries to swallow you each day. It will be the life preserver that turns your dreams into reality.

- **Self-esteem**. If your life is exciting, you eat to live. When it's not, you live to eat. If you have low self-esteem, you'll sit on the couch eating an industrial sized bag of Milk Duds just to break up the monotony of your life. Now is the time to turn your back on such self-defeating behavior and seize the stimulating life that is waiting for you.

- **Self-respect**. When you don't like yourself, the need for immediate gratification takes over and translates into comfort eating. Immediate gratification is the devil licking his chops. He's the bakery for the overeater, the casino for the gambler, the singles' bar for the person who needs a one-night stand to feel wanted. Learn to respect yourself enough to recognize the repercussions of that sinful morsel before the devil gets you in his grasp.

- **Self-confidence**. If you don't think you're worthy of achieving your dreams or just being happy, you will always come up short. You have to learn that you're worth more than letting fifteen minutes of chewing and swallowing negate your daily exercise.

- **Self-worth**. If you had a machine that spit out a $100 bill every hour, how would you treat it? You'd polish it, make sure it had the best fuel, keep it in a safe environment and make sure nothing could harm it. You wouldn't leave it uncovered outside so it could rust, would you? Do you treat yourself as well as you would treat that $100 bill machine? If not, it's time you realize that you need to treat your body like the precious machine that it is.

- **Self-discipline**. Your body is just like a computer. You can program it to say "no" to temptation. It may take more than a few reboots to get the "no" chip up and running, but programming your body to say "no" is vital and one of the most rewarding steps along the way.

- **Self-improvement**. The No. 1 reason most people say they overeat is boredom. As you may have heard before, "there are three types of people – those that make things happen, those that watch things happen and those that wonder what happened." If you go through the same robotic, monotonous, predictable routine every day, you will do self-destructive things just to break up the boring daily pattern. Self-improvement will eliminate boredom. Self-improvement is permanent and eliminates the need for immediate gratification. So what type of person do you want to be?

Americans are always looking for a quick fix to make their problems go away – pills to ease their depression, a fad diet that promises miraculous weight loss, trendy treadmills to transform their bodies. But there are no quick fixes to remedy long-term-behavior. You may feel for a while, or drop a few pounds, but until you address the inherent reasons that created your current situation, the changes will be temporary. Think of your body like a computer. You can't have the life you want until you program yourself to change your behavior in a way that leads you to a fulfilling and exciting life.

Once you get your holistic foundation programmed and aligned, it will be the catalyst that lights the round to increased self-esteem, self-respect, self-confidence, self-worth, self-discipline and self-improvement. There isn't going to be a magic moment when the clouds part, the sun shines into your window, and a voice says, "Now is the time to make your life better." It's all up to you. Start by creating good communication with yourself. How well do you know yourself? It's time to reflect on who you are, where you are going, and what you want your life to be about. Get on a path and assess who you are. If you take it in small and attainable steps, in the end you'll like the person you are talking to.

You will create a new best friend in yourself.

YOU control tomorrow. If you really want to change your life, stop blaming your problems on your mother, your father, the person who discriminated against you, the friend who rained on your parade during your formidable years, the bully who hit you in fourth grade, or the teacher who didn't pay enough attention to you. Even if there are things that were traumatic in your life, they are over now and can't be changed. You've had time to mourn and rehab yourself. You can give birth to a new you and have a relationship of total communication with yourself. Every effort and action you take from now on will make you self-destruct or self-improve based on the things you do.

Your body doesn't come programmed with this information. Like anything, it's built and learned over time. There are two reasons people don't do something – they don't have the information, or they have the information and choose to ignore it. this book will give you the knowledge to change your behavior. Once you make all the pieces fall into place, anything will be possible for you. Self-esteem will build self-respect, which creates self-confidence and leads to more self-worth, self-discipline and self-improvement. You will have that life preserver firmly in hand, and it will be up to you to create an exciting life and realize your dreams. Knowing that you are worth the effort to make the changes that will allow you to realize your dreams can become as life-affirming and automatic as a heartbeat. But it all starts with you. You control your destiny. What path are you going to choose?

Are you ready to meet your new best friend?

1
Getting started

Remember the saying, "You are what you eat?"

Think about that. You don't want to be as lethargic or inactive as a cow, do you? When was the last time you saw a cow galloping off into the sunset with sweat dripping from its brow? A cow isn't what we want to be. So why do we keep eating those burgers? Put down the bacon unless you want to feel like a pig. If one of the goals you hope to achieve after reading this book is losing weight or building a better body, it all has to start with nutrition. As we learned in the introduction, eighty percent of how we look is what we eat, so you know that now. it's up to you to either act on it or ignore it.

How much are you overweight? Ten pounds? Twenty pounds? More? What if I told you I would give you a beautiful necklace made of the most pure gold in the world? You would like that, wouldn't you? But what if I told you that as pendants on that necklace, you would have to wear a ten-pound bowling ball for every ten pounds you are overweight? Think about those extra twenty pounds as two bowling balls hanging from a chain around your neck, because that's the extra baggage that you're making your body carry around every day. Think of how difficult it would be to go to the mall, work, walk, sleep or make love with two ten-pound bowling balls hanging from your neck. Even with no exercise, your routine daily tasks each day would require a Herculean effort. Yet that's the added pressure you put on your heart, back and joints every day when you're carrying around an extra twenty pounds. But think about how good it would feel when you finally got rid of those bowling balls. Besides reducing your risk for heart diseases, disc problems or a future hip replacement, you'd feel great, wouldn't you?

The first step you have to take in order to lose those heavy bowling balls and get on the road to a better body is to refuse to be a victim to our weight-obsessed society. What you weigh is just gravity to Earth. While weight is an important and valuable way to measure improvement and progress, what's more important is lean muscle and how much of your body is made up of fatty tissue. Muscle weighs more than fat, so one pound of muscle is going to have much less mass than one pound of fat. So measure your percentage of body fat and try to improve on that. A simple guideline is this: a normal man's body fat should fall into the 14-23 percent range, while women should shoot for 17-27 percent. These percentages are for the ideal body, based on not accepting mediocrity in your life. You are worth more than being mediocre.

Lowering your body fat starts with nutrition because you've already learned that eighty percent of what you look like is what you eat. To prove my point, look at the nearest gym. There are aerobic instructors who have just as much cellulite in their butt as some people who never work out. All the cardiovascular workouts in the world won't stop fatty deposits from covering your body if you eat the wrong foods. Some people rationalize their poor diet by saying, "I exercise all the time. I can eat whatever I want." So they vacuum a party size bag of Doritos or a large pizza for dinner and can't figure out why they still don't feel comfortable when they look in the mirror or try on bathing suits.

The first step to lowering your body fat percentage is to have a realistic plan. Without it, most people fall into a pattern of losing, then gaining. It's unrealistic to think you're going to go from flabby to fit overnight. If you fail to plan, you plan to fail. Remember, there are no magic pills to make your dreams come true. You have to set realistic goals and keep the four components of a holistic life in alignment. At the same time, you have to build self-esteem, self-respect, self-confidence, self-worth, self-discipline and self-improvement.

The road to better health starts with a simple formula. Your percentage of body fat goes up or down based on the amount of fat and sugar you take in. Your percentage of body fat will never go down if you're eating food soaked or fried in 100 percent fat. The math never adds up. You have to isolate foods in your diet that are high in fat and sugar and try to eliminate or limit them.

How do you do that? Follow these formulas:

Computing a healthy FAT INDEX

Before you buy a food product, look at the total number of fat grams and calories listed on the label. You can compute the FAT INDEX by following this formula: Total number of fat grams X 10 ÷ number of calories per serving = Fat index.

For example, in an energy bar containing 6 grams of fat and 200 calories per serving, you would compute its FAT INDEX as follows:

6 X 10 ÷ 200 = .3 or 30%.

Is that a healthy FAT INDEX? No! A healthy level should be no more than .2 or 20%. Any food item that is more than 20% fat should be extremely limited or eliminated from your diet if you need to lower your percentage of body fat. If you do not maintain a healthy body fat percentage, you increase the risk of developing heart disease and diabetes.

Computing a healthy SUGAR INDEX

To compute the SUGAR INDEX, follow the same formula:

Total number of sugar grams X 10 ÷ number of calories per serving = Sugar index.

For example, in that same energy bar containing 23 grams of sugar, you would compute its SUGAR INDEX as follows:

23 X 10 ÷ 200 = 1.15 or 115%.

You should strive for a SUGAR INDEX that is also less than 20%, so the sugar level in the energy bar is woefully unhealthy. Sugar and fat create the same fatty tissue on the body. So "fat-free" means nothing if there is still too much sugar in the product.

When selecting foods in the grocery store, you should choose only products that have a FAT INDEX and SUGAR INDEX both less than .2 or 20%. My Cardinal Rule for weight loss is to only eat foods that satisfy both formulas. And if you obey my Cardinal Rule, you will take weight off and keep it off.

You have to study those labels. Just because you buy something in a health food store, it doesn't mean it's healthy. Here are a few examples of foods and how they stack up using the fat and sugar formulas.

- **Ultra Slimfast French vanilla drink**. Has 220 calories per serving with 3 grams of fat and 35 grams of sugar.

    Fat Index: 3 X 10 ÷ 220 = .14 or 14%

    Sugar Index: 30 X 10 ÷ 220 = 1.59 or 159%

    This drink, despite its claims that it will make you thinner, is pure sugar. Since fat and sugar both increase your percentage of body fat, this product will do nothing to help you lost weight and keep it off.

- **Kraft Fat-Free Shredded Cheddar or Mozzarella Cheese**. Has 40 calories per serving with 0 grams of fat and 0 grams of sugar.

Fat Index: 0 X 10 ÷ 40 = 0 or 0%

Sugar Index: 0 X 10 ÷ 40 = 0 or 0%

I put all my patients on Kraft Fat-Free Pre-shredded Mozzarella or Cheddar Cheese. They can spread over a salad, put it in a sandwich, over broccoli and don't have to worry about adding any fat or sugar to their diet.

- **Jenny Craig Nutritional Meal Bar**. Has 210 calories per serving with 5 grams of fat and 20 grams of sugar.

Fat Index: 5 X 10 ÷ 210 = .24 or 24%

Sugar Index: 20 X 10 ÷ 210 = .95 or 95%

The label on this product reads, "Tastes Great! Lose Weight Naturally," but it fails both the fat and sugar test. You might as well be eating a candy bar.

- **Pure Protein energy bar**. Has 280 calories per serving with 5 grams of fat and 4 grams of sugar.

Fat Index: 5 X 10 ÷ 280 = .18 or 18%

Sugar Index: 4 X 10 ÷ 280 = .14 or 14%

This satisfies both the fat and sugar formulas. So if you're looking for a meal replacement bar, skip the Jenny Craig and go for a Pure Protein.

- **Organic Colorado Cracked Wheat Bread**. Has 120 calories per serving with 1 grams of fat and 4 grams of sugar.

Fat Index: 1 X 10 ÷ 120 = .08 or 8%

Sugar Index: 4 X 10 ÷ 120 = .33 or 33%

If the name of this product doesn't sound healthy, I don't know what does. But when you run it through the formulas, it satisfies the Fat Index but when it comes to the Sugar Index, it fails. If it doesn't satisfy both formulas, skip it.

- **Sugar-free Snackwell shortbread cookies**. Has 130 calories per serving with 5 grams of fat and 0 grams of sugar.

  Fat Index: 5 X 10 ÷ 130 = .38 or 38%

  Sugar Index: 0 X 10 ÷ 130 = 0 or 0%

  Millions of people are snapping up products like this so they can have their snacks but also feel like they're eating something that's better for them. While this product satisfies the sugar formula, it fails the fat formula. Don't eat them.

- **Newman's Own Unsalted Pretzels**. Has 110 calories per serving with 1 grams of fat and 1 grams of sugar.

  Fat Index: 1 X 10 ÷ 110 = .09 or 9%

  Sugar Index: 1 X 10 ÷ 110 = .09 or 9%

If you want a snack, this is one that's good for you because it satisfies both the fat and sugar formulas. Another healthy snack is this: take a brown paper lunch bag, thinly coat the bottom of the bag with popcorn kernels, roll it up and pop it into the microwave for two minutes. You'll have fresh, hot popcorn without using any oils. Skip the butter and salt and you've got yourself a healthy snack at home or at the office.

One thing to keep in mind when you're looking at the labels is what type of sugar is used. Most companies just glop the sugars together and call it a sugar gram. They don't tell you that you're getting sugar from chocolate chips like you would if you were sucking down cookies. You'll want sugars that are natural derivatives from fruit or fruit pastes, not sugar like you'd get in a Snickers. Look for natural, fruit-derived sugars, or natural fructose.

When you hit the grocery store next time, buy only products that satisfy both formulas and you'll be on your way to losing weight and keeping it off. It might be hard at first, you might need to carry a calculator, you might need to pass up some of your favorite items, but it will be worth it. the Fat Index and Sugar Index is powerful information that will arm you to wage war against unhealthy eating. You have the knowledge now, are you going to use it or ignore it? You know you're worth it, so start using it.

Need more ammunition? Here are some rough guidelines to help you improve your diet and eliminate some of the sugar and fat you're eating:

Don't fall victim to "fat-free" marketing. A lot of companies call their products fat free, but all they do is cut the fat and double up the sugar content. You're going to gain the same weight because fat and sugar create the same body fat. So study those labels. The sugar content in Ben & Jerry's Lowfat Chocolate Fudge Brownie rises to 30 grams from 27 grams of sugar in the standard Chocolate Fudge Brownie. Likewise, the sugar content in fat-free Campbell's Cream of Chicken Soup doubles from the regular version. And "reduced-fat ham?" What they don't tell you is reduced from what to what? Did they put the pig on a treadmill? No way! You can cut off the corner of a slice of ham and call it "reduced fat." Don't let labels fool you.

- **Avoid foods high in fat**. If you really want to lower your percentage of body fat, you cannot be soaking and drowning and saturating your food in mayonnaise, butter, margarine and cooking oils. They're almost 100 percent fat. If you have to use oil, use virgin olive oil, canola oil or grapeseed oil. It's still 100 percent fat, but at least it cleanses your arteries instead of clogging them.

- **Skip the soda.** Suppose that I told you I had a mystery drink that I was going to force you to drink. If I described it as something that could take the paint off a building and rust off a car battery terminal, would you drink it? No way. Yet people guzzle down liters of soda every day. There isn't one food source in soda. It's just chemicals in a can.

Replace red meat with fish as often as possible. Would you rather eat a big hunk of slothen animal that's shot up with growth hormones to fatten it up in a hurry, or something that spends its life swimming and being active 24 hours a day? Which do you think would be healthier? The only exercise a cow gets is when college kids get drunk and tip it. It's best to limit or eliminate red meat from your diet. But if you switch to fish, don't bread the fish in bleached-white flour and drown it in greasy oil. If you do, you're a magician. You just turned the fish into a cow.

- **Avoid foods high in additives, preservatives and chemicals.** If God invented it, go ahead and eat it. If man invented it, don't trust it. God did not invent Cheese Whiz or Cocoa Krispies. Stick a Twinkie on the counter next to your phone and come back in twenty years. They'll both still be in the same place with the same consistency because both were made from chemicals, not from food. The thing that's killing Americans is we have too much processed food in our diet. Nature produces food that's good for you. If man made it, chances are he used chemicals to extend its shelf life so corporations and grocery stores can maximize profits. You never hear a hunter say, "Honey, I'm going to hunt for processed meat." We shouldn't be walking down grocery store aisles hunting for it either. The body only recognizes food that comes naturally. It doesn't recognize chemicals. So unless you want to be a science project, stop eating processed food.

Don't let your environment control you, you control your environment. Schools are providing less and less physical education and more and more unhealthy, fattening foods in their cafeterias. Hospitals dispense large quantities of fried and high-caloric food in their cafeterias, while their beds are filled with obese patients who suffer from heart disease and diabetes. Schools are supposed to educate children and hospitals are supposed to be informative and healing, but both provide self-destructive and hypocritical methods of food consumption. And grocery stores aren't doing anything to help, either, creating cereal aisles packed with boxes of garbage that are 99% sugar, addicting children to unhealthy eating habits.

- **Invest the time needed to plan and prepare healthy food to consume daily.** Many people who are alone say to themselves, "It's not worth cooking if it's just for me." Even if it is just for yourself, you are worth all the time and effort it takes to do *anything* that will create a better life. Pamper yourself, take the time to prepare nutritional meals. We're talking about your life. Our society has become lazy in terms of food preparation. Recently while at a supermarket, I saw a frozen turkey and cheese sandwich that was marketed as "Just need to microwave and eat." I laughed. We can't even slap two pieces of bread together and make a sandwich? That's too much work? Your body is worth more than feeding it a nuked frozen sandwich. You should only want the best fuel to keep you moving and alive, so take the time to prepare meals that are nutritionally sound and enjoyable.

- **Create the right attitude and commitment so winning results will follow.** Do not ever say to yourself that you will "try" to follow the instructions and nutritional guidelines of this book. If you do, you will fail. Do you "try" to brush your teeth or do you brush your teeth? Do you "try" to shampoo your hair or do you shampoo your hair? Follow everything in this book with commitment and a new enthusiasm, and you will win. But you have to stop trying and start doing.

Take in most of your calories early in the day. Do you gas up your tank before the trip or after the trip? Americans do it backwards – skip breakfast, scarf down lunch, and then vacuum the refrigerator all night, at a time when they're going to be the least active. Give your body time to burn off the calories instead of loading up at night when you're going to be sedentary. Gas up the car *before* the trip. Have a big breakfast, a moderate lunch, light dinner and no solid food within three hours of sleep. And if you say you skip breakfast in the morning because you're not hungry, I bet it's because you're overeating at the fridge before bed. Let me lock you in a closet at night and let you out in the morning. I guarantee you'll magically be hungry by morning. You'll probably be gnawing on my ankles when I let you out.

That's enough to get you started. Incorporating any one of these guidelines into your daily routine is going to put you one step closer to developing the self-esteem, self-respect, self-confidence, self-worth, self-discipline and self-improvement you'll need to build the ring of life that will create more excitement and fulfillment. You know you are worth taking this information and running with it. the ball is in your court now. it's up to you to use the knowledge or ignore it.

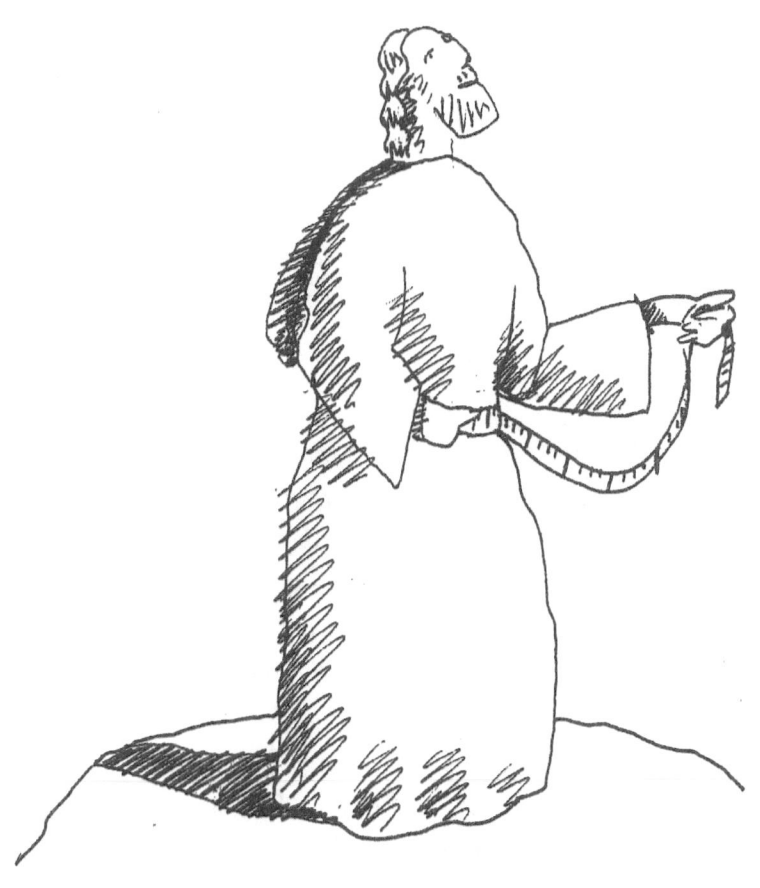

Illustrations by Robin Brisker

RB.

2
Self-esteem

Remember the first car you bought for yourself? It was so exciting. You were so proud of that car. You'd wash it all the time, put in premium gasoline, take it in for regular maintenance checks. You took great care of it because it had value to you. But after a while, it became like everything else. The novelty wore off, so you didn't wash it as often, and didn't care anymore what kind of gas you put in it. You just accepted that it was your car and would be there for you. But what happens eventually? The car breaks down, doesn't it?

We do the same things with our bodies. There are times we take care of it, feed it healthy fuel. But then – more often than not – we feed it junk. We don't maintain it. we don't take any pride in ourselves or our bodies because we don't have the self-esteem to care. And when you lack self-esteem and stop caring about your body and it's daily upkeep, eventually it's going to break down just like that old car you stopped caring about. But there aren't any NAPA Auto Parts stores to replace your body. There aren't any trade-ins available. You have to work with what you have.

We have to start recognizing that our bodies are our most precious possession. Aren't you worth feeding your body the best fuel and maintaining it regularly? We don't have to accept apathy when it comes to our own bodies. We can turn our old '59 Chevy of a body into a Ferrari. But it's all up to you.

If you had a best friend that made promises to you at the beginning of every week and broke all of them by the end of the week, how long would that person be your best friend? How many times have you promised yourself, "Starting on Monday, I am going to eat right and exercise," and "Starting on Monday, no more chocolate, beer, or pizza?" But Monday never comes. In order to build self-esteem, you have to be able to trust yourself. Make commitments you will keep. When you make a promise to yourself, be able to "take it to the bank." Then, your newly developed best friend will not go away.

To build self-esteem, keep in mind the four categories that create a holistic and balanced life – nutritional, physical, emotional and spiritual. Are there areas that are weak in your life and which lead to low self-esteem? Are there areas that you're strong in, and that you could use to build up other areas? To start building your self-esteem, ask yourself these questions:

1. Does it make me uncomfortable when someone compliments me?

2. Does it make me uncomfortable when someone buys me an unexpected gift?

3. Do I save my best clothing for special occasions?

Do I find it difficult to think that people will automatically like me or accept me? If you answered "yes" to any of those questions, you need to work on your self-esteem. You have to realize that you are worthy of receiving compliments, of being surprised by a gift; of wearing clothes that make you look your best all the time and not just on special occasions; and that you can be recognized for the good person you are just by being yourself. To build self-esteem, you will need to realize your goals. Start by making two lists:

What five qualities do I possess that make me feel the best about myself?

    1.

    2.

    3.

    4.

    5.

What five things would I like to change about myself?

    1.

    2.

    3.

    4.

    5.

To start feeling like YOU are worth saying "no" to that hot-fudge sundae or that YOU deserve to walk into the gym and make a change. Take one minute each day to read over the positive qualities you wrote down on the first list. Take a minute to pat yourself on the back for those good qualities you already have. Think about ways you can strengthen and build on them. Then, take one minute each day to read over the things that you want to change.

Is there a way to use your positive qualities to improve your weaknesses, and then eventually be able to erase them from the list of things you'd like to change? Remember, as much as we want to believe it's possible, there are no overnight solutions. You have to start by setting attainable and measurable goals. If you want to lose weight, is it realistic to lose one-eighth of a pound a month? Of course it is. It may not sound like a lot, but think about it this way: If you lost one-eighth of a pound every month, you would eventually disappear. If you lose just one-eighth of a pound every month, your weight is going in the direction you want it to go – DOWN! – and at least you're not gaining more. That's an accomplishment within itself. If you want to exercise more, is walking one-hundred yards a day a realistic goal? Of course. If that's more than you're doing now, that's a good thing. It's a step in the right direction. Before long, losing one-eighth of a pound each month or walking one-hundred yards each day won't be enough for you. You'll realize that your body is more important than the immediate gratification you get from the sugar-coated Crisco you eat from the middle of an Oreo cookie. You'll feel the power to push yourself. You'll raise the bar because you'll realize that YOU'RE worth it.

Won't that feel great?

3
Self-worth

Most people take better care of their possessions than they do their own bodies. A perfect example is a guy down in San Antonio who came to me for nutritional counseling. I asked him to tell me about his daily diet.

"I always start out my day with a good breakfast," he told me. "I love a big breakfast."

"That's good," I told him. "It's best to take in most of your calories early in the day to give your body time to burn them. What is your typical breakfast?"

"Usually a breakfast burrito," he said. "My favorite is tortilla, eggs and bacon."

"What do you do with the grease after you cook the bacon?" I asked him.

"I usually save it to cook other meals because it adds a nice flavor," he said. "If I already have enough to cook with, I pour it into a can, let it harden and throw it away."

"Why don't you just pour it down the sink?"

He looked at me like I was crazy.

"Because it would plug the pipes!" he exclaimed. "So what you are telling me is that you are worried about bacon grease plugging up an inch-and-a-half steel pipe that can be replaced for a few dollars, but you have *NO* problem thinking it will sail right through microscopic arteries in your body without eventually clogging them, too? What you're saying is that you care more about the plumbing in your kitchen than your own body?"

The guy's jaw dropped and he looked me in the eye.

"My God," he said. "I never thought about it like that."

That, more than anything else, is the reason why no matter what fad diet you try, what exercise program you start, what job you have or what relationship you enter, you will almost always fail in the end if you don't treat yourself at least as well as the pipes in your kitchen. If you don't think you're worth the effort it takes to look good and feel good, you might as well keep pouring grease down your pipes. Who do you fear more – a plumber working to unclog a kitchen drain, or a cardiologist who says you need surgery to unclog blocked arteries? With stints or eventually even a pacemaker?!

There are other things many of us do to ourselves that are just as self-destructive as pouring grease down our pipes. If a man reads a warning from the surgeon general that says smoking will kill him, and he keeps lighting up the cancer sticks, there should be red flags all over the place that that person desperately needs to work on his self-worth. If a woman is spending money on something she knows will shorten her life, what should that tell her? If it's more comforting to sleep than to be awake; if you would rather have your eyes closed where it's dark, instead of open so you can see the light; if you'd rather retreat than participate in fun activities, these should be a red flag that tell you that your life isn't exciting enough. You need to realize that your life IS worth separating yourself from self-destructive behavior. If all the red flags you are given still don't program in that "no" computer chip, you need to find a way to reboot. You need to reassess the value of staying alive. It's time to do whatever it takes to make the changes needed to turn your dreams into reality and to be a participant in life and not a watcher. After all, you're worth it!

To build self-worth, always keep in mind the four categories that create a holistic and balanced life – nutritional, physical, emotional and spiritual. Are there areas that make you feel worthy of realizing your dream and others that make you feel unworthy of living the life you want to live? To start building the self-worth you need to turn your dreams into reality, ask yourself this:

What five qualities would I want an ideal mate – the one I want to spend the rest of my life with – to possess?

1.

2.

3.

4.

5.

Look over the list. Study it. Now, ask yourself – and be totally honest – which of those qualities do you possess that would make you an ideal mate for yourself? So many of us demand honesty and sincerity from our ideal mate, but we're often not honest or sincere with ourselves. We join a gym, but never go. We tell ourselves that we'll lose weight, but never do. We tell ourselves we want to have a better job, but never take the classes or develop the skills and knowledge needed to get that job. We make New Year's resolutions that we know we are never going to fulfill. We must be honest with ourselves. If we can't be honest with ourselves, how can we expect the same from a mate? It's no wonder so many people have an intense fear of being alone. It's because they lie to themselves. Whenever you tell yourself you want to do something and then never do it, you're lying to yourself. And who wants to be stuck with a liar? Not you. You deserve better than that.

It's time to find a new best friend in yourself, to feel worthy of realizing your dreams, to feeling you're worth *not* pouring that bacon grease down your pipes. If you want to be worthy of being your own best friend, don't lie, deceive, undermine or procrastinate when it comes time to improve your life. If you were in a job and told your boss repeatedly that you'd do something and then never did it, how long would you last? You would never lie to the people you respect, so stop lying to yourself.

To get to the level of self-worth that you deserve, take one minute each day to read over the list of qualities you want in your ideal mate. Does your behavior match those qualities? If it doesn't, do one thing every day to change your behavior and make yourself worthy of being your own best friend. When you do that, give yourself a pat on the back and feel proud of yourself. Don't ever let anyone else tell you that you can't do something. Don't let anyone set limits on you. You can do anything you want to do, because you are worth it!

4

Self-confidence

Have you ever met anybody who ascended into Heaven, came back to Earth and showed you family slides?

Have you ever met someone who went to Hell and came back with family photos?

Well, if the answer to those questions is "no," that means you've never met anyone who is better than you or anybody who is worse than you. You are just as good as anyone else, and it's time you realized that. You don't have to envy someone else's house, spouse, body, or occupation. With determination and effort, you can turn your dreams into reality, too. You should feel worthy of building the qualities that the people you respect have. You should realize that until you have the self-confidence to feel worthy of turning your dreams into reality, you will always be a dream and never a doer. You have to stop looking at others and telling yourself, "I would love to be in a relationship or have a friendship with that person, but they would never be interested in me," or, "I would love to have that job, but I could never get it." How do you know? It's time to stop writing the end before the story even starts. Remove the limits that you've placed on yourself and reprogram your computer.

I remember a group of obese women for whom I was providing nutritional counseling. I advised them to exercise to get the physical part of their life in alignment with the nutritional aspect they were working on. Well, these obese women took an aerobics class, lost a little weight through healthier eating and really started to feel good about themselves. They still had a long way to go, but they were so enthusiastic and passionate about taking control of their lives that the aerobics teachers couldn't even keep up with them. So you know what I did? I let these obese women start teaching aerobics classes in the health facility. Their self-confidence soared as they reached out and helped others get on the road to health. They started telling their students when they were worried about their regressing instead of progressing. The wheels of these instructors became aligned – the nutritional and physical metamorphosis made their lives more exciting and by helping others, they suddenly had purpose. They started by taking one small step at a time, and they reprogrammed themselves to believe that with hope, anything is possible, even going from obese to teaching aerobics classes.

You have to believe in yourself. If you don't, who will?

To build the self-confidence you need to turn your dreams into reality, ask yourself these questions:

1. *If there's an event that requires competition or training, do I feel like I have the ability to win? Do I feel I possess the ability to earn someone's support?*

2. *When I see good qualities in someone, can I see the same qualities in myself?*

3. *Is self-improvement easily attainable for me?*

When you can answer "yes" to each of the four questions, you have a healthy amount of self-confidence. This will help you build that holistic life preserver of "selfs" that will give you self-empowerment to accomplish any goal. If you've answered "no" to any of these questions, take one minute each week to review the answers. What have you done in the last week to improve your self-confidence? What have you done in the last week that makes your life exciting? What have you done in the last week to improve yourself? What have you done in the last week to ensure that the four categories that create a holistic life – emotional, spiritual, nutritional and physical – are in alignment?

Take just one minute each week to review your answers until you answer "yes" to every question.

Once you are able to do that, you'll be a person who feels worthy of turning your dreams into reality. You will be brimming with self-confidence because you're worth it. And there is absolutely nothing wrong with telling yourself, "I love myself for what I just did."

You deserve everything you accomplish. You *should* feel excited about it.

5
Self-respect

When I was in college, I worked in a deli. Every night before I went home, the owner made sure I cleaned the meat slicer thoroughly because he respected what that machine meant to his business. Soon, I respected it, too.

"Make sure before you leave tonight to open up the machine, clean the blade, make sure everything is spotless, and then turn the engine light off," my boss ordered me. "That way, when we come in tomorrow morning, it's smooth, and it works good every day. That's what you've got to do."

So every night, I would clean the blade, make sure there wasn't a scrap or fiber of food on it, turn the motor, off, and let the machine rest so it would be ready to go the next day.

But we rarely treat ourselves with the same respect. Before we go to bed, we scarf down ribs and frat-house-party-sized bowls of butter-soaked popcorn while we watch other people participate in activities on television – sports, movies, game shows. So all night, our body is like a Vegamatic, churning and working to digest the food we ate before going to sleep. And, then we wonder why we feel tired the next day. We haven't respected ourself enough to keep the machine clean, let the body rest and start the next day clean and ready to go.

It's time to respect yourself enough to make sure your machine is ready to go the next day.

To build self-respect, keep in mind the four categories you must keep aligned in order to create a holistic and balanced life – nutritional, physical, emotional and spiritual. Do this exercise:

Rank the ten people you respect the most:

1.

2.

3.

4.

5.

6.

7.

8.

9.

10.

Now, ask yourself this question:

Where would you rank yourself on that list?

If you didn't rank yourself at the top of your list, write down the qualities of the people whom you respect. Do you respect someone who maintains a healthy diet? Who exercises regularly? Who has a great job? Who has great focus? Who has great ambition? Who has a great relationship? Who gives back to the community? Who is great at achieving goals? Take one minute each day to review the list and ask yourself, "What am I doing to change my behavior so I will possess the qualities enveloped by the people I respect?" By taking just one minute each day to remind yourself of your ideal image, you may stop yourself from doing one small thing that makes you dislike yourself. If you catch yourself doing something self-destructive, or disrespecting your machine, modify your behavior to earn your own respect. Pretty soon, you'll catch yourself exhibiting those qualities you admire in others, and you will be a step closer to turning your dreams into reality.

6
Self-discipline

One of the things that always make me laugh is when someone comes to me for nutritional counseling, but attaches conditions to any program of self-improvement I want them to follow.

"You can give me any nutritional plan you want," one guy said to me, "but you can't take away my beer. I love my beer and you can't take it away."

"I'm not taking away your beer," I told him. "One beer a night is fine. You just have to drink in moderation."

"Well, what if I don't drink any beers during the week and save them up?" he asked. "I can go out on Saturday night and drink a six-pack, right?"

I tried to think of a way to explain his flawed reasoning, and this is what I said:

"What if I told you that I'm going to stop brushing my teeth during the week? Monday through Friday, I'm not going to brush my teeth. But on Saturday, I'm going to brush the hell out of them until my gums bleed. Think that would be OK?"

The truth is, self-discipline is something that we need to exercise every day if we want to turn our dreams into reality. Americans are enamored with the thought of quick-fix solutions because the quick-fix eliminates the need for self-discipline. Want to lose weight? Take a pill. Want to gain weight? Take a pill. Can't go to the bathroom? Take a pill. Go to the bathroom too much? Take a pill. We pay personal trainers billions of dollars a year to count repetitions for us. What happened to self-discipline? There is no way jumping on an exercise machine for three minutes a day is going to make you look great. I don't care what the beautiful model on TV tells you. It's never going to happen.

The only way you're going to turn your dreams into reality is to work at it, step by step, day by day, until good behavior becomes as ingrained as the bad behavior once was. Remember, the self-discipline chip doesn't come programmed in your body. You have to program it over time, and occasionally when you get a virus that affects the "no" chip, what you have to do is reboot.

To build self-discipline, keep in mind the four categories that create a holistic and balanced life – nutritional, physical, emotional and spiritual. Are there areas where your self-discipline is weakest? Are there areas and skills where you exhibit strong self-discipline that you could use to strengthen weak areas? Build self-discipline by asking yourself these questions:

1. *Do I feel I'm more productive if someone else has me programmed to do something? Do I accomplish more when someone else directs me or when I set my own agenda?*

2. *Is it comforting to feel dependent on others?*

3. *Would I rather be an actor in someone else's play, or my own playwright?*

Honestly assess where you stand in relation to self-discipline. Review the list of qualities you would see in an ideal mate and the qualities

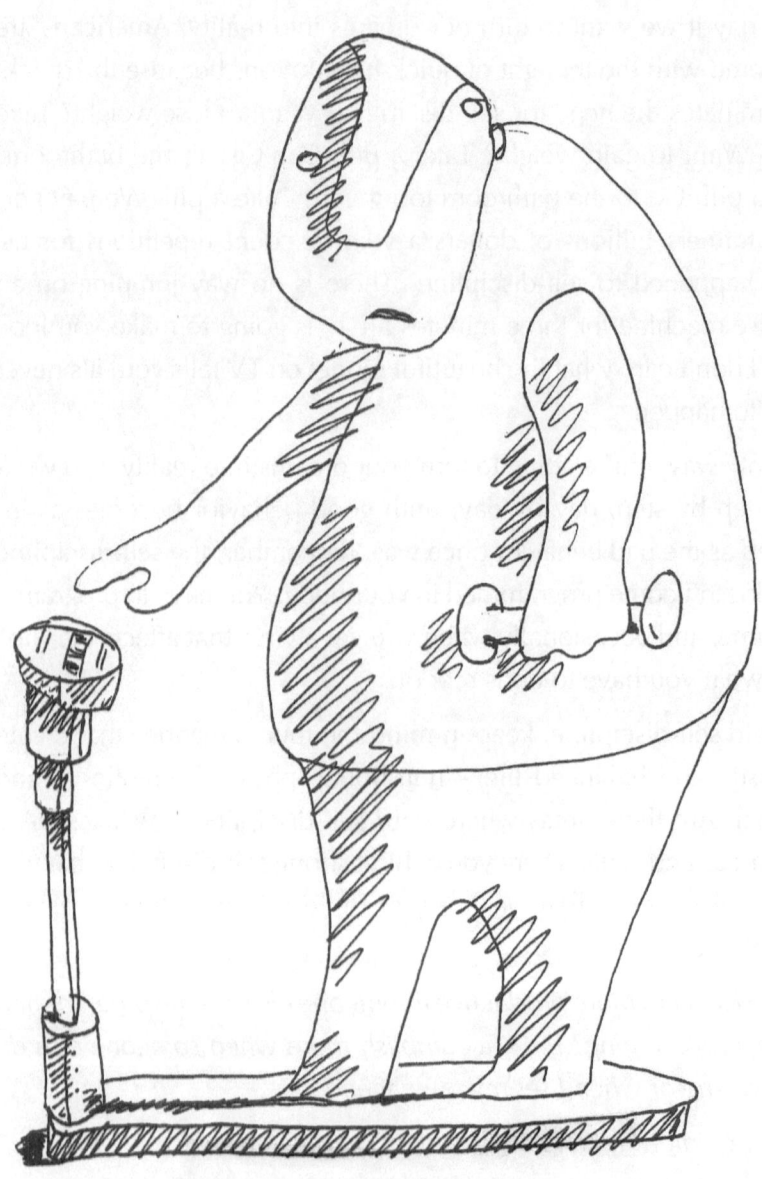

Illustrations by Robin Brisker

enveloped by the people you respect. Take a minute each day to examine the self-discipline you've shown or the self-discipline you've lacked relative to building those qualities in yourself.

Then make another list:

What five things do I need to improve on?

1.

2.

3.

4.

5.

Realize that there are no quick-fix solutions. There are no pills you can take to modify your behavior. Too often, people who want to get in shape or lose weight look in the mirror and see themselves, then look in a magazine and see Cindy Crawford and say, "Screw it, give me a beer."

You don't have to do that. You can turn your dreams into reality if you just exercise the self-discipline and knowledge that you're worth it. You've got to get excited about the prospect of a new you. Do you need to reboot the computer? Is the "no" chip working. Is the "I can" chip working? If they aren't, reprogram yourself – bad habit by bad habit, day by day. You don't have to be one of those people who say, "Wouldn't it be nice if…" or, "My life would be better if I could just change…"

Be a doer not a dreamer.

Look over the list of five things you want to improve and ask yourself, "What have I done in the last month to improve in that area?" Modify your behavior to improve those areas and you will build self-discipline. Practice using the "no" chip to resist the wrong foods, keep using the "yes, I can accomplish anything I put my mind to" chip until you don't have to reboot as often. If you don't program those "no" and "yes" chips correctly, you will forever be on the roller-coaster ride of weight loss and weight gain, getting fit then becoming unfit and discouraged. Just like an alcoholic can't drink on special occasions, you should never allow occasions or give into immediate gratification that may compromise your self-discipline. As convenient as you think it is, the only thing fast food is going to do is destroy self-discipline fast. Use that "no" chip. If it's not working, time to reboot.

You're worth the effort.

7

Self-improvement

One of the most rewarding experiences I've had in my thirty years of nutritional counseling centers around a 295-pound suicidal man who was directed to me after all methods of support failed to help him. He had been to medical doctors, psychiatrists and even his priest. When he came to me, he was on twelve different medications for his health and psychological problems, and he had a huge chip on his shoulder. He made it clear he didn't like the doctors, didn't like the priest and was prepared to not like me. I asked him why he had a problem with the doctors.

"They told me what *they* thought I had to do," he said. "But they never asked one question about me. They didn't care about me as a person."

So over the course of the next few weeks, I quizzed him about himself. I asked about the events in his life where he thought things turned for the worse, when sadness started to overshadow happiness, and when food became more pleasurable than living an exciting life.

Finally, I asked him, "Did you ever feel focused enough in life that when you woke up in the morning you knew you would have a good day?" "No," he said.

"Do you know how much power you have to control your destiny?" I asked. "The doctors and your priest are not your sole or soul providers to help you develop independence. They can navigate the ship only if it's ready to leave the dock. It's up to you to decide if you're ready."

Suddenly, his eyes brightened, the weight of the world lifted from his shoulders.

"You're right," he said. "I don't need them, do I?"

"No, but here's what you do need," I said. "You have to quit blaming other people if you're going to keep eating the amount of food that creates an uncomfortably overweight person. Who are you going to blame tomorrow after you and I develop a nutritional plan? Who are you going to blame then for eating too much?"

He was silent. But he realized that the person he saw in the mirror every morning was the only person who could tell him how much food to eat every day. He knew it was up to him to control his weight, control his eating and take control of his life.

"You *don't* need doctors or your priest or even me to survive. But we can be a strong support system to help you as long as we have your best interests at heart," I said. "Do you think I have your best interests at heart?"

"Yes."

This person was ready to kill himself when he came in to see me. When he walked in the door that first time, he wanted to die. The *last* thing he cared about was eating properly. But once he realized he controlled his own destiny, once he was ready to change, once he realized he had the ability to modify his behavior and turn his dreams into reality, he was ready to go to work. It was his first experience with self-empowerment.

"I want you eating one big healthy plate of food, no second helpings,"

I told him. "And I want you to get your butt out of the chair and do things that make your life exciting."

He dedicated himself to losing weight. He stumbled once in a while, but he learned that it takes time to program that "no" chip. He kept rebooting and eventually developed the self-esteem, self-worth, self-respect, self-confidence and self-discipline to drop his weight from 295 lbs. down to 175 lbs.

About a year and a half after he first walked into my office and after he lost the weight, he came for a visit and dropped into a chair across from me. He looked stunned.

"Do you know what I just did?" he asked.

"What?"

"I rode my bike all around town for four hours," he beamed.

"Four hours?"

"Do you know *why* I rode my bike around town for four hours?" he asked.

"No. Why?"

"Because I could," he smiled. "I haven't been able to ride a bike since I was a kid. My legs rubbed together. I couldn't fit on the seat. But I don't have to worry about that anymore. I *RODE* a bike! I haven't felt this good in so long that I don't want it to stop."

What he realized is that everyone needs a positive release to a negative feeling in order to improve. All the psychiatrists in the world could have told him, until they were blue in the face, that he was worth the effort it took to change his life. But until *he* took responsibility for himself, their words had no more meaning than a Hallmark card. Once he took responsibility for himself and started getting his wheels aligned, all the "selfs" came together. His self-esteem, self-worth, self-respect, self-confidence, self-discipline and self-improvement solidified around the four categories that create a holistic life – nutritional, physical, emotional and spiritual – and created a life preserver that saved his life. His healthy eating allowed him to be more physical, and the happiness he felt gave him purpose. He liberated himself and removed those bowling balls from around his neck.

And so can you.

To make sure you are effectively improving yourself, make the following lists:

What are five things that would make my life more exciting?

1.

2.

3.

4.

5.

What five things have I always wanted to accomplish, but never did?
1.

2.

3.

4.

5.

Here's the litmus test: Have you ever run into an acquaintance you haven't seen for a couple of months and been asked, "Hey, what's new?"

If you ever answered, "Nothing," or, "Same old stuff," it's time for a change. You have to create a life that's so exciting that when you run into that person, you'll have a laundry list of exciting things you've done that will make them green with envy. There must be a book you've always wanted to read, class you wanted to take, activity you wanted to try, place you wanted to visit, language you wanted to learn, or instrument you wanted to play. Take one minute each week and ask yourself what you've done to make your life more exciting or what you've done to move toward accomplishing one of your goals. When you accomplish one goal, cross it off and make another. Tell yourself how proud you are of what you've accomplished. Don't wait for others to recognize your gains.

If you have an addictive personality – and a lot of overweight people do – take advantage of it. Everyone needs a release from the stress and pressure of work, home and family.

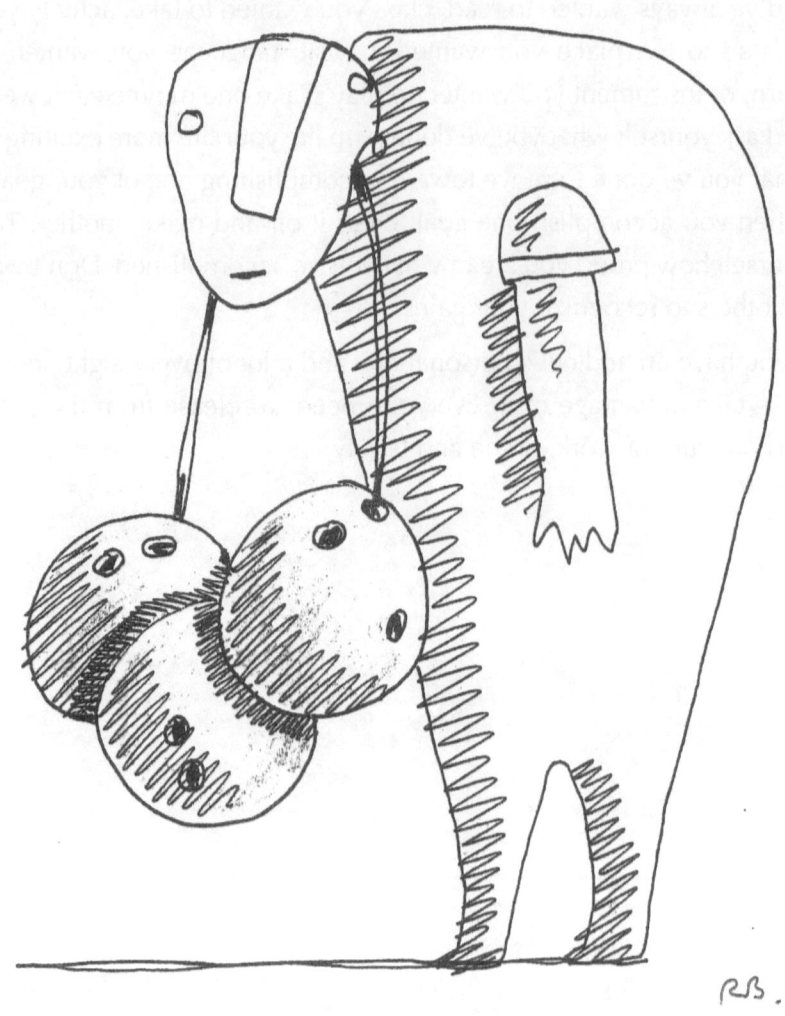

Illustrations by Robin Brisker

The release can't be the consumption of food, betting on a football game or the numbing of your senses from alcohol. Those should be red flags that your "no" chip needs to be rebooted. Instead of seeking a release through self-destructive behavior, find releases that will improve you, give you the green flag to a happier life, and focus your addictive personality on self-improvement. Read that book you've wanted to read. Take that class. Try that activity you wanted to try. Visit the places you want to visit. Learn the language you dreamed of speaking. Start that exercise program you've always put off. Being addicted to anything other than self-improvement can be self-destructive. And think how exciting it could be to be addicted to self-improvement.

There are no limits on how much you can improve. The only person who can set limits on you is you. Lose the bowling balls. You'll look great.

It's time to turn those dreams into reality.

8

Living the lesson

The most powerful feeling that you will experience is the same thing that enveloped that 295-pound suicidal man before he turned his life around: self-empowerment. It is that feeling of knowing that there's nothing stopping you from turning your dreams into reality. It's the knowledge that you are omnipotent and possess the self-confidence and self-discipline to accomplish any goal you set your sights on. It's the pride of knowing that you have the self-esteem and self-worth to refuse to let anyone rain on your parade.

We live in a society that's designed to build dependency. We're told we need to take a pill to control something we don't understand. We're told in order to lose weight we *have to* stay on the latest fad diet. We're told if we want to get into shape we need to join a gym or hire a personal trainer. Why? If we don't have a personal trainer, does that mean we can't work out? If we don't have someone plan our eating program like Jenny Craig with boxed lunches, does that mean we're going to gain seventy pounds and burst? Do you want to live your life dependent on someone else to tell you what to eat? Of course not, because you have developed self-empowerment. You have the ability to be independent and self-sufficient. You know you have the power to turn your life around, to modify your behavior and turn your dreams into reality. You know how to go to a grocery store and pick foods that are nutritionally sound and will keep the nutritional aspect of your holistic life in alignment.

You also know that self-empowerment takes a lot of work. We have to rely on ourselves for reminders that there are no quick-fix solution. There are no pills that burn fat by doing nothing. There are no machines that produce washboard bellies just by rolling up and down on the floor with it for three minutes a day. Turning any of your dreams into reality takes much more than three minutes a day. It takes building that ring of life – self-esteem, self-worth, self-confidence, self-respect, self-discipline and self-improvement. There is no immediate fix. There are no immediate results. Remember immediate gratification is just the devil licking his chops, waiting to pounce at the precise moment your computer needs to be rebooted.

You have to make sure you maintain your machine and keep it running smoothly so it needs fewer and fewer reboots. Everything that involves self-empowerment involves a graduation of some form of system that you develop within yourself to be independent to everything around you. Then by graduating from each chapter of this book, you will have developed that life preserver, that ring of self-empowerment that will change your life.

Now that you know you're worth the effort to make the lifestyle change needed to get to a healthy weight and maintain it, you are ready for Brisker's 10 Commandments for Weight Loss. Tear the next page out. Stick it to your refrigerator. Make copies and hang them above your desk, on your mirrors, in your cupboards, on your dashboard, because living the rules outlined on this one-page sheet will make you lose weight and keep it off: **Brisker's MINDSET Healthy Responses for Weight Loss**

I. THOU SHALT NOT EAT THESE FATS:

Butter

Margarine

Mayonnaise

Cooking oils

II. THOU SHALT NOT EAT THESE SUGARS:

Candy

Cakes

Pies

Sodas

Cookies

Canned fruits

Canned vegetables

Ketchup

III. THOU SHALT EAT THESE MEATS SPARINGLY:

Beef

Veal

Pork

Lamb

Hot dogs

Sausage

Bacon

Processed meats

IV.Thou shalt limit salts:
Allowed 155 mg per day

V.Thou shalt limit alcohol:
Allowed 1 glass of wine (Cabernet, Merlot, Chardonnay, Chablis) or 1 lite beer per day

VI.Thou shalt eat fresh fruits:
2-3 fruits per day and juice counts as a fruit.

A serving is the size of your fist.

VII.Thou shalt eat fresh vegetables:
5-7 fresh or frozen vegetables per day.

A serving is the size of your fist.

VIII.Thou shalt eat these proteins:
2-3 protein items per day (chicken, fish, turkey, seafood, soy products, lentils, beans, peas, protein shakes, protein powers, egg whites, ion-exchange edamame, fatty acids and omega-3)

IX.Thou shalt limit carbohydrates:
Only 1 of the following 6 grains and starch items per day:

1. 2 slices of bread (must be rye, wheat, pumpernickel, 9-grain, 12-grain or oat bran).

2. 1 bagel (rye, wheat, pumpernickel, 9-grain, 12-grain or oat bran).

3. Oatmeal or cereal that satisfies both the Fat Index and Sugar Index.

4. Brown Rice only

5. Sweet Potato only (baked, boiled, steamed or grilled, not fried).

6. Pasta (must be <u>semolina</u>).

<u>X.THOU SHALT DRINK LOTS OF WATER</u>
64 ounces per day:

<u>BRISKER'S CARDINAL RULE:ALL FOODS MUST SATISFY FAT AND SUGAR FORMULAS</u>
Number of fat grams X 10 ÷ calories per serving < 20% or too high in fat

Number of sugar grams X 10 ÷ calories per serving < 20% or too high in sugar Here is a more in-depth explanation of each of Brisker's 10 Commandments for Weight Loss, along with some other guidelines to follow:

Fats

Some fat in your diet is necessary to create the essential fatty acids the body requires to absorb fat-soluble vitamins – Vitamin A for the immune system, skin and lungs; Vitamin D for bone growth; Vitamin E for the heart; Vitamin K for natural blood clotting. Those healthy fats can be found in fish and nuts. The key is to avoid the fats that are bad for you like those typically found in fried foods. Avoid anything that is hydrogenated or partially hydrogenated.

And read those labels. If a product lists in its ingredients, "one of the following oils is used…" which you see in most candy bars, what it really means is that they're buying the cheapest bulk oil so they can to turn the biggest profit and clog your arteries. Canola oil, virgin olive oil and grapeseed oil are more expensive, but they don't clog the arteries. Find products that use them.

Also, don't fall for the "fat-free" or "lowfat" or "reduced fat" marketing gimmick that makes food manufacturers billions of dollars while we keep getting more and more overweight. They tell you they cut the fat grams, but they don't tell you they added a zillion grams of sugar, enough to rip the teeth out of your mouth. You're still going to raise your percentage of body fat and gain the same weight because sugar grams create fat the same, if not more, than fat grams. Eating a fat-free chocolate cake may make you feel less guilty than eating a fat-*full* chocolate cake, but it shouldn't. You're going to gain exactly the same weight so you should feel exactly the same guilt.

Bottom line: A healthy nutritional plan does not include butter, margarine, mayonnaise, unhealthy cooking oils, or anything hydrogenated. Get the fats your body needs from healthy sources like fish, nuts or avocados. Buy only products that pass the FAT INDEX test.

Fresh fruits and vegetables

What would you do if a friend called you with this dinner invitation?

"Hey, I would love to have you over for dinner tonight. It will be great. I've got some six-month-old food I'm going to serve, and I'd like you to join me."

Would you go? Why not? We eat six-month old food all the time and don't think twice about it.

Think about a can of peas. First, the peas are grown with pesticides and quick-growing chemicals, then they're picked and spend a couple of days on a truck before they end up at a factory. There, they're treated with more chemicals and preservatives and end up in a can. The can of peas sits in the factory warehouse for a while before it's shipped to a distribution warehouse where it sits for a couple of months, then sent to a grocery store warehouse and sits again for God knows how long. Finally, it ends up in a grocery store where it's rotated onto the shelves. Six months after those peas were picked, we buy them, stick them in our cupboards and eventually eat them.

What if you bought fresh peas that were picked the same time as the canned peas? Say you put them in your refrigerator. What would the peas look like after six months? Your refrigerator *crisper* would be your refrigerator *rotter*. They'd be mush. But we eat six-month old food every day without batting an eye. Why not go three aisles down and buy fresh vegetables? We eat canned food all the time and wonder why the cancer rate is so high. The more we mess with Mother Nature, the more we chemicalize food, dye foods and process them, we become a walking chemistry and paint set and that means more trouble down the road. My feeling is that a lot of the different types of cancer from the intestines, colon, and prostate comes from the processed foods we're putting into our bodies. The more natural we eat and the more we get back to juicing and eating fruits, grains, and vegetables that are full of antioxidants which prevent cancer, the more we're going to maintain a healthier lifestyle with fewer mood swings and a lower cancer risk.

Bottom line: A healthy nutritional plan allows 2-3 fruits per day, with juice counting as a fruit. If you have a choice between a fruit or its juice, always eat the fruit. There will be more folic acid, more Vitamin C, more fiber and less sugar. If you have juice, it *has* to be 100% unsweetened, preferably fresh squeezed. If you have a banana, have it only in the morning. The only fruits you can have after 4 p.m. are melons, berries or grapefruit because they are high in water and low in fructose.

A healthy nutritional plan allows 5-7 vegetables each day. However, don't let any of those fruits or vegetables be canned. Only fresh or frozen. How do you know if a frozen vegetable is healthy? Simple. If you buy frozen spinach, look at the ingredients. It should say "spinach" and that's it. the only ingredient in a frozen fruit or vegetable should be the fruit or the vegetable. Also, steer clear of frozen vegetables with sodium or BHT. A portion of fruit or vegetable should be the size of your fist.

Sugars

Because sugar grams create the same fatty tissue as fat grams, it's important to avoid foods high in sugar, just like you avoid foods high in fat. Read the labels on the products you buy. Most food manufacturers just glop the sugars together and call it a sugar gram. They don't tell you that you're getting the same sugar you'd get if you were scarfing down chocolate chip cookies. Look for products with sugars that are natural derivatives from fruit or fruit pastes, not sugar like you'd get in a Snickers.

Bottom line: A healthy nutritional plan does not include foods with high sugar contents like candy, cookies, cakes, pies, soda, canned fruits and vegetables, and ketchup. Buy only products that pass the SUGAR INDEX test. Get the majority of your sugar grams from fresh fruit. If you're looking for a natural sugar substitute, the only one I recommend would be Stevia.

Meat and protein

Protein is vital to a healthy diet because it helps build lean muscle. But get the protein your body needs from healthy sources like chicken, fish and beans.

Hot dogs, sausage, bacon and processed meats are soaked in preservatives that some studies say may cause healthy problems. On top of that, the fat content in those items will put you over the amount needed for a healthy diet.

Remember how we said that we want to feed our machine only the best fuel to keep it running smoothly? Consider this: After a butcher takes out the "good stuff" and ships it to the grocery store, he's left with pig lips, pig brain, pig eyes and pig parts that he sticks into a blender with chemicals and makes a "protein shake" that he squirts into a casing that resembles a prophylactic and calls it a hot dog. While there are exceptions and there are probably acceptable hot dogs on the market, we know that it's best to eat food God created. Obviously, God didn't come up with the concept of the hot dog. So why risk it when we know the fuels that God created will keep our engine running efficiently? You have the knowledge, now it's up to you to either use it or ignore it.

Bottom line: A healthy nutritional plan includes protein from chicken, fish, turkey, seafood, soy products, lentils, beans, peas, egg whites, and protein powders that satisfy the FAT INDEX and SUGAR INDEX formulas. You should have two or three protein servings each day. Preferred meats and fish should be either baked, broiled, boiled, grilled or steamed. Limit the amount of beef, veal, lamb, pork, hot dogs, sausage and processed meats in your diet.

Grains and starches

The most important thing to remember when dealing with the starches in your diet is to avoid drowning the bread and potatoes in butter and margarine. It's fine to enjoy a couple of slices of bread each day, but like everything else, moderation is the key. Only having one of the following six items per day is a great jump-start to taking the weight off. Once you get to your healthy weight, you may be able to have two of the items per day, but not until you achieve your target weight and are on a maintenance plan. **Bottom line:** A healthy nutritional plan incorporates ONLY ONE of these six items in a daily diet:

1. 2 slices of bread (rye, wheat, pumpernickel, 9-grain, 12-grain or oat bran).

2. 1 bagel (rye, wheat, pumpernickel, 9-grain, 12-grain or oat bran).

3. Brown Rice.

4. Sweet potato.

5. Pasta (best to be Semolina). Sauce must satisfy the fat and sugar formulas.

6. Oatmeal or Multi-grain cereal that satisfies the fat and sugar formulas.

Salts

We know that salt retains water, which causes us to bloat and puff and makes the rings get tight on our fingers. We also know that when we're trying to firm up and lose weight, what's the first kind of weight we're going to lose? Water weight. So every time we put extra sodium on our tongue, it's like saying, "I want to delay my weight loss for as long as possible. I don't want to get to the fatty tissue. I just want to keep losing the water in my body that's bloating me so I never get to the fatty tissue." So in order to burn the fatty tissue which results in a lower body-fat percentage and more firmness, we have to limit our salt intake.

Bottom line: A healthy nutritional plan allows 155 milligrams (mg) of salt intake each day. Read the labels. Avoid foods high in sodium. Limit the amount of salt used to season food.

Alcohol

Alcohol can be a great social function as well as helping with digestion, thinning the blood and helping cleanse the arteries. It's also good because it relaxes the system. One glass a day will help take the edge off. But that doesn't mean you can brown-bag it in the parking lot. Where most people mess up with alcohol is when they transition into needing alcohol to numb out their life. Remember the characteristics you listed for your ideal mate? Did the list include overindulging and drinking too much? We don't want someone who needs to numb themselves to communicate with others or lacks the self-discipline to resist the temptation of immediate gratification. Even if problems arise, if you drink to numb yourself and think your troubles will be swept away, think again. Use self-improvement, not alcohol to eliminate your problems.

The big excuse I get from people who break Brisker's 10 Commandments for Weight Loss by drinking more alcohol than the plan allows is, "I take clients out and they drink," or, "I'm going to a party and they're going to be drinking." If you feel uncomfortable in these situations, here's what to do: Take the glass of wine, divide it into thirds and add two-thirds club soda with a twist of lemon or lime. That way, you can have three drinks and you have only consumed a single glass of wine. You didn't' break the Fifth Commandment.

Bottom line: A healthy nutritional plan can include one glass of wine or one lite beer each day. No mixed drinks or hard liquors are allowed.

Water

One of the most difficult things I've encountered while doing nutritional counseling is convincing people to drink enough water each day to strengthen antibodies and the immune system. I could never understand why people wait until they have mucus dripping out of their nose and have a throat that's so sore they can't even talk before the light bulb goes on and they say, "Hey, I should be drinking more water and juice."

The water you drink is like a human oil change. What happens to your car if you don't change the oil? It breaks down. The same thing will happen if you don't flush your system out with water every day. It gives bacteria the opportunity to grow, it gives chemicals in the food we eat to deposit and cause health problems. We need to flush our system every day with water. If we don't, the body will break down, just like the car that never has its oil changed.

Bottom line: A healthy nutritional plan includes 6-8 eight-ounce glasses of water each day.

Caffeine

What would happen if I told you to go outside every morning, start your car, put it in park, floor it and keep it like that for thirty minutes? How long do you think that car is going to last? That's what we do every day we drink more than one cup of coffee. We get our heart rate racing, but we're not moving. The body says, "Shouldn't I be running or taking an aerobics class or walking to get my heart rate this fast?" Just like the car that has its gas pedal floored but isn't going anywhere, your body will break down before long.

One cup of coffee a day is fine. It can regulate you, it can get you to go to the bathroom consistently and help you get started in the morning. But if you need more than one cup a day to keep you going, you're a speed freak. You need to find something exciting to get you jump-started instead of needing something external.

Bottom line: A healthy nutritional plan can include one cup of coffee a day, but anything more is a risk. In addition to caffeine, avoid foods that contain other stimulants, such as ma Huang, ephedrine, garanja, and willow bark extract, all found in many energy bars, alleged fat-burning pills or drinks.

Vitamins

In order to get all the vitamins and minerals you need to stay as healthy as possible, you might have to eat twenty-eight meals a day. If you do that, you might as well stamp Goodyear on your butt. So each person should take a good multivitamin every day.

To illustrate the need for a good daily multivitamin, look at insects. They get tons of antioxidants that build strong antibodies because they live off the land. This enables them to fight off the germicides and pesticides that we spray on plants. In the meantime, we eat the vegetables that are sprayed with the germicides and pesticides, or eat so much processed food that we don't get enough antioxidants. And we wonder why the cancer rate is so high?

We need to take Vitamins A, C, and E every day, which are collectively our antioxidants. To do it completely right, take a multivitamin with A, C and E in the morning with your breakfast. In the evening, you'll have depleted all your C and E, so take an extra C and E with your dinner and you'll have a perfect balance of antioxidants for the day.

In addition, as we get older, men need to make sure they get zinc on a daily basis to lower their risk of developing prostate cancer and women need to take calcium with magnesium to lower their risk of developing osteoporosis.

Dairy

If you really feel the need to have some dairy in your diet, almond milk or fat-free, sugar free yogurt products for the probiotic consumption are acceptable.

Also acceptable is Kraft Fat-Free Shredded Cheddar or Mozzarella Cheese, which I talked about in the second chapter, because it contains no fat or sugar grams. Frozen yogurt, that is all natural, fruit-sweetened or stevia sweetened is a great dairy product also for daily consumption. Beware: Many dairy products in the United States have hormones, steroids, or even anti-biotics in the products we are purchasing today......obviously very unhealthy!!

When to eat

Timing of when you eat is just as important as what you eat. We already know it's most important to have a big breakfast, to fuel up at the start of the trip, not after you run out of gas. If a banana is one of the fruits in your diet, it should only be eaten in the morning because it's high in carbohydrates. That banana should be part of your gasoline that keeps you energized over the course of your daily events.

Why do you need to fill up with energy before you go to sleep? Fruits that can be eaten at night are the high-water, low-sugar fruits – melons and berries. They make perfect snacks in the evening. Apples, oranges, pears and peaches should be eaten in the morning or afternoon and not at night because they are higher in sugar.

It takes up to three hours to digest vegetables, fruits, chicken and fish. It takes a *lot* more time to digest dairy products because of the lactose and red meat because it is high in cholesterol and fat. So it's important if you eat red meat – and I recommend that you don't – that you eat it in the afternoon so it doesn't make your stomach do somersaults all night while you're trying to rest.

Bottom line: No solid food within three hours of sleep.

Serving size

One of the biggest misconceptions we have is misinformation regarding the "minimum daily requirements" for vitamins, proteins, carbohydrates, calories and everything else. Every person is different in terms of activities, what they do during the course of their day and what they need to consume to satisfy their daily routine. How can a marathon runner who runs 26 miles with their heart rate over 100 beats per minutes have the same "daily requirements" as someone who sits at a desk all day and answers the phone? So it's silly to try to fit everyone into the same cookie cutter by saying we all have the same "minimum daily requirements." We don't. Every individual is as unique as their DNA. That's why some people can eat a large pizza, drink a keg of beer and still look thin, while as Richard Simmons jokingly said, "another person can eat a bag of M&Ms and wake up in the morning with Ms on their ass." But there's good news and bad news. The bad news is that you might not have a high metabolic rate, and you may not be one of the people who are blessed to burn off everything they eat. But the good news is that if you do have a slow metabolic rate, it can be changed. For every pound of fat that you change into muscle, you burn fifty more calories a day. When you change fatty tissue into lean muscle mass, you're changing your body into a more efficient calorie-burning machine. The flip side is that for every pound of lean muscle you let atrophy into fatty tissue, you store an extra 50 calories a day. So you can change your machine and rejuvenate the body to give yourself a better metabolic rate. You may never get an ideal metabolic rate that lets you burn everything you eat, but if you change a pound of fatty tissue into a pound of muscle, you'll burn an extra fifty calories daily by doing nothing. So, if you convert two pounds of fat, that's one-hundred calories. Bottom line is hope, and you have some control over your metabolic rate.

It's up to you. You have the knowledge now. Are you going to use it or ignore it?

People are always asking me about quantities, "How many calories should I eat a day?" We don't want to get into calorie-counting because it's counterproductive to what we've been working on in this book – behavior modification. The most important thing is to get the "no" and "yes" chips programmed properly. The only lesson we have to learn is when to get up from the table. Get a plate and fill it with one protein item, a couple of vegetables, a fruit, get something to drink and enjoy the meal. Then, guess what? Get up from the table and go do something exciting. You're done eating. If you ask to have something passed and put more things on your now empty plate you're just going through the motions because you're *not* hungry. You're just chewing and swallowing. If you're still asking to have things passed every day like it's a Thanksgiving Roman orgy, there's a void in your life. Stop yourself, get up and find something exciting to do to fill that void. You must create a lifestyle that embraces good nutrition so it becomes as life-affirming as breathing. The trying is over. It's time to start *doing*. You don't *try* to brush your teeth. You don't *try* to wash your hair. You just do it. The same should be true for healthy eating.

To show that you don't have to deprive yourself or starve yourself, here is a sample menu for a month. This isn't a diet, it's a collection of meals that are very colorful, very creative, using no oils, no fats, no margarine, and nothing is fried or sautéed. This menu follows Brisker's 10 Commandments for Weight Loss and has helped hundreds of people I've worked with lose thousands of pounds and keep them off because each meal is conducive to losing weight or maintaining a healthy weight. I promise that if you follow this menu; obey my Cardinal Rule of making sure the foods you eat satisfy the Fat Index and Sugar Index formulas; and follow Brisker's MINDSET for Weight Loss, you will lose weight in a healthy and permanent way. Just like in life, there will be times that you break the Commandments. The key is to limit those stumbles and balance those mistakes by getting right back to your nutritional plan. **Week 1 sample menu**

SUNDAY
Breakfast: Ham and asparagus quiche; mixed fresh fruit.

Lunch: Green salad; orange. When eating a salad, use only lemon and vinegar or balsamic vinegar dressing.

Dinner: Baked Portobello mushroom stuffed with crab, red pepper and no-fat cheddar cheese; steamed spinach.

MONDAY
Breakfast: Protein shake. When blending a protein shake, use a protein powder with less than one gram of fat and one gram of sugar per serving and use only fresh or frozen fruit and fresh-squeezed orange juice.

Lunch: Chicken and vegetable quesadilla; pear.

Dinner: Baked cod; spinach and rice squares; steamed carrots.

Breakfast: Shredded wheat with blackberries.

Lunch: California rolls; steamed vegetables.

Dinner: Chicken chowder; spinach salad; watermelon.

WEDNESDAY

Breakfast: Protein shake with mixed berries. **Lunch:** Turkey breast; stewed tomatoes.

Dinner: Grilled halibut; small green salad; pineapple.

THURSDAY

Breakfast: Scrambled egg whites with spinach and onion; half of a whole wheat English muffin; mango and kiwi.

Lunch: Turkey breast wrap – slice of deli turkey wrapped around lettuce, onion and tomato; pear.

Dinner: Greek salad with fat-free feta cheese, onions, black olives, tomato and cucumber; mixed blackberries and raspberries.

FRIDAY

Breakfast: Oatmeal with dried cranberries.

Lunch: Half of a grilled chicken breast; raw vegetables – celery, broccoli, cauliflower.

Dinner: Crab cakes; grilled yellow peppers and onions; grilled potato slices; watermelon.

SATURDAY

Breakfast: Protein shake.

Lunch: Tuna salad on pumpernickel; apple; carrot and celery sticks.

Dinner: Grilled chicken with pineapple teriyaki glaze; grilled Portobello mushroom; grilled asparagus; honeydew melon. **Week 2 sample menu**

Sunday
Breakfast: Mexican frittata with egg beaters, cilantro, tomato, onion and fat-free cheddar cheese; mixed melon.

Lunch: Half a turkey sandwich in a whole wheat pita with lettuce and tomato; orange.

Dinner: Boneless and skinless chicken thighs stuffed with minced onion, carrots and leeks, braised in reduced Merlot with basil and garlic; mashed potatoes and parsnips; steamed yellow and green squash.

Monday
Breakfast: Protein shake with strawberries.

Lunch: Fat-free ham on rye with onion, lettuce and tomato; yellow and red pepper strips.

Dinner: Spinach salad with water chestnuts, red onion and cilantro; gazpacho.

Tuesday
Breakfast: Cheerios with half of a banana.

Lunch: Cold plate – chicken, raw vegetables, pickles, strawberries.

Dinner: Baked falafel with cucumber yogurt sauce; assorted relishes – olives, radishes, celery, peppers; frozen green grapes.

Wednesday
Breakfast: Protein shake with papaya.

Lunch: Grilled chicken; small green salad.

Dinner: Tortilla pizza – no-fat cheddar cheese, grilled peppers, mushrooms and onions grilled on a no-fat tortilla green salad.

THURSDAY

Breakfast: Shredded wheat with blueberries.

Lunch: Cold grilled shrimp on greens, cherry tomatoes and celery sticks.

Dinner: Baked chicken; roasted vegetables – carrots, onions, zucchini, red pepper; small green salad.

FRIDAY

Breakfast: Protein shake with half of a banana.

Lunch: Tomato basil soup; raw vegetables.

Dinner: Seafood risotto – mussels, shrimp, salmon; steamed asparagus and carrots; spinach salad with yellow and red peppers.

SATURDAY

Breakfast: Pancake with apple-blueberry sauce.

Lunch: Chicken chowder; small green salad.

Dinner: Grilled mahi with grilled pineapple salsa steamed carrots and snow peas; grapefruit and orange sections.

Week 3 sample menu

SUNDAY

Breakfast: Protein shake with mango.

Lunch: Lettuce wrap with shrimp, Napa cabbage and bean sprouts; fresh pineapple.

Dinner: Grilled chicken breast with garlic and orange juice marinade; steamed zucchini and squash; cold asparagus salad.

Monday
Breakfast: Breakfast burrito in a fat-free whole wheat tortilla with scrambled egg whites, onion, cilantro and salsa fresca.

Lunch: Chicken salad on greens; grapes.

Dinner: Grilled shrimp; broccoli salad with onions and dried cranberries; grilled yellow squash.

Tuesday
Breakfast: Protein shake with peaches.

Lunch: Half of a whole wheat pita with grilled ahi tuna, lettuce and tomato.

Dinner: Grilled turkey breast cutlets; grilled asparagus and mushrooms; grilled fresh pineapple.

Wednesday
Breakfast: Fat-free, sugar-free zucchini muffin.

Lunch: Cream of broccoli soup; small green salad; peach.

Dinner: Scallops kabobs with yellow peppers, onions and mushrooms; brown rice salad with asparagus and carrots; strawberries.

Thursday
Breakfast: Protein shake with raspberries.

Lunch: Half of a veggie sandwich on rye with lettuce, tomato, onion, cucumber and bean sprouts; dill pickles and radishes; strawberries.

Dinner: Turkey breast meatloaf; barley salad with asparagus, onions and mushrooms; steamed carrots and snow peas.

Breakfast: Shredded wheat with blackberries.

Lunch: Shrimp spinach salad with orange juice dressing; orange.

Dinner: Filet mignon; half of a grilled sweet potato; grilled onion slices; strawberries.

SATURDAY

Breakfast: Protein shake with mango.

Lunch: Chef salad with fat-free cheddar cheese and fat-free ham.

Dinner: Grilled ahi tuna with teriyaki marinade; grilled yellow and red peppers; kiwi and raspberries.

Week 4 sample menu

SUNDAY

Breakfast: French toast (made with Egg Beaters); orange and grape-fruit sections.

Lunch: Potato leek soup; green salad.

Dinner: Grilled chicken with lime juice and tequila marinade; spinach salad with red onion and orange sections; grilled zucchini and summer squash.

MONDAY

Breakfast: Protein shake with strawberries.

Lunch: Salad with red peppers, cucumber, broccoli and onion with oil and vinegar dressing (use only half-teaspoon of olive oil); 2 crackers with no fat cheddar cheese.

Dinner: Grilled salmon; half of a grilled sweet potato; grilled yellow and red peppers.

TUESDAY

Breakfast: Oatmeal with skim milk and raisins.

Lunch: Grilled chicken breast on salad greens with vegetables; raspberries and cantaloupe.

Dinner: Grilled pork tenderloin; sauerkraut with apple and onions; steamed carrots and cauliflower.

WEDNESDAY

Breakfast: Protein shake.

Lunch: Half of a whole wheat pita with turkey, lettuce, tomato, cucumber and bean sprouts; orange.

Dinner: Grilled salmon; pasta primavera with asparagus, carrots, onions, mushrooms, tomato and basil; sliced tomatoes.

THURSDAY

Breakfast: Cheerios with half of a banana.

Lunch: Cold grilled chicken; salad with cherry tomatoes, red onion and cucumber.

Dinner: Tuscan bean casserole with white beans, onions, butternut squash, spinach and fresh tomatoes; spinach salad; strawberries.

FRIDAY

Breakfast: Protein shake with strawberries.

Lunch: Vegetable soup; small salad; orange.

Dinner: Grilled chicken fajita with grilled vegetables and tomato slices.

SATURDAY

Breakfast: Egg white omelet with spinach, red onion and fat-free cheddar cheese; cantaloupe.

Lunch: Cajun grilled chicken open-faced sandwich; raw vegetables – radishes, carrots, snow peas.

Dinner: Grilled halibut with mango salsa; broccoli salad; half of a grilled sweet potato.

If there's one thing I hope you take away from this book, it's the realization that there isn't a panacea. There isn't one program that fits all, or one diet or exercise program that will change the lives of everyone who tries it. The only thing that fits all is self-empowerment – the life preserver you create for yourself when you achieve symmetry between the nutritional, physical, emotional and spiritual elements that create the person you are. Each person is a snowflake with different shapes, markings and curves that distinguish it. The holistic ring you create when you build self-esteem, self-worth, self-respect, self-confidence, self-discipline and self-improvement is the only program that will always turn your dreams into reality. without this, you will fail every time.

Here is one final test. Many of us try to live a good life so that after we die, we can go to a better place, to heaven. Answer the following questions: *What are five characteristics or life style qualities I hope heaven possesses?*

1.

2.

3.

4.

5.

Now, ask yourself this: What is preventing me from having those things *NOW?* What can you do to create a utopian life for yourself now? It can happen. You have the knowledge now to turn your life around. Are you going to use it or ignore it?

The day can come when the four categories of your holistic life will fall into perfect alignment. You will have developed the self-esteem, self-worth, self-respect, self-confidence, self-discipline and self-improvement needed to turn your dreams into reality. You'll look into the mirror and revel at the qualities of your new best friend – you! The feeling of self-empowerment will be overwhelming, and you will feel so much pride that you'll want to shout. The unspoken words that create that moment will sum up a lifetime spent searching and working towards love, acceptance and accomplishment. Your dreams will have arrived.

It will be heaven on Earth.